Second Degree
Reiki
Manual & Journal

Second Degree Reiki
Manual & Journal

A Practitioner's Innovative Guide to Healing Life Events

Eleanor Haspel-Portner, Ph.D.

Second Degree Reiki Manual & Journal
Eleanor Haspel-Portner, Ph.D.

Copyright © 2024 Noble Sciences, LLC.

All rights reserved.
This book or any portion thereof may not be reproduced or used in any manner whatsoever without the express written permission of the publisher except for the use of brief quotations in a book review.

ISBN:
978-1-931053-09-9
978-1-931053-10-5

Other titles by Eleanor Haspel-Portner
First Degre Reiki Manual
Cosmic Guidance for Mastering Your Life
Cosmic Secrets
Astrology Essentials
*Marriage in Trouble: A Time of Decisio*n

Author's websites
www.nobleenergywellness.com
www.DrEleanor.com
www.moptu.com/DrEleanor

Illustrations created by
Eleanor Haspel-Portner, Ph.D and Cindy O. Smith
Book Design by Michelle M. White

*Dr. Mikao Usui & Mrs. Hawayo Takata
brought Reiki to us in its pure form.*

*We carry it with light, love, and integrity
honoring its pure tradition.*

Contents

Foreword
1

Introduction
5

How to use this Manual & Journal
13

The Reiki Treatment and Hand Positions
16

How to Do a Second Degree Reiki Treatment
47

Developmental Treatments
55

Treating Yourself Structurally
105

Dreams
141

About the Author
145

Collaborative Assistance
147

Classes
149

♦ ♦ ♦

Illustrations

Illustration 1: All Three Second Degree Reiki Symbols 47

Illustration 2: Hon Sha Ze Sho Nen 49

Illustration 3: Sei He Ki 50

Illustration 4: Cho Ku Rei 51

Illustration 5: Mrs. Takata's Drawing of Second Degree
  Reiki Symbols 53

Steps for Doing a Second Degree Reiki Treatment 54

Ilustration 6: Annotated 64-Gate Mandala 107

Illustration 7: The Hindu Chakra System 108

Illustration 8: The Tree of Life 109

♦ ♦ ♦

Foreword

Shortly after I began the practice of Transcendental Meditation in January 1974, I began having experiences that I could not explain with my scientific mind. I was already a clinical psychologist and in training as a Jungian Analyst, so when I began having dreams about knowing with a "K", I was open to receiving new awareness. Nevertheless, I was a bit surprised when my first "big" energy experience occurred. At the time, I was sitting quietly when I suddenly experienced a brilliant light coming toward me. I gasped in awe as the light's brilliance surrounded and enveloped me. My awareness opened, activating and expanding my understanding and knowledge of the universe and of consciousness.

Many shifts in my consciousness continued. I remembered seeing auras from the time I was born, and I began to reclaim my psychic gifts while working with clients. Then, during my first trip to the Los Angeles area in August 1976, I recognized that the area around Pacific Palisades was my true home. Shortly thereafter, I decided to relocate my home, family, and private clinical psychology practice there. As I was preparing to move in June 1977, I was told by a colleague to check out a healing modality called Reiki. I took his advice and had the great fortune to attend a First-Degree Reiki class with Mrs. Hawayo Takata, who brought Reiki from Japan to the western world, in attendance. Thus,

I heard Mrs. Takata tell her story and learned directly from her about her experiences using Reiki.

The first night after my first Reiki experience, I treated my head positions using Reiki energy. The following morning, I awoke and immediately noticed that I could see without putting on my glasses. This convinced me that Reiki was a real healing modality, since my myopia was so severe at that time that I could not even see the face of a person standing three feet away from me. So, seeing clearly across a room and seeing street signs at a distance proved to me that something very profound had happened from my Reiki experience and treatment.

As I understand it, Reiki is a white light energy transmitted from Master to student in the "oral" tradition of the past. Reiki initiations are always done in person or at a distance using a formula handed down through generations from master to student. The activation of the energy in a student is done according to a formula that imprints the Reiki symbols and their energy into the student's aura or energy field.

A student, once initiated by a Reiki Master/Teacher, is imprinted with Reiki energy in their auric field for their lifetime. Reiki energy then automatically activates in their hands whenever they touch any living thing, including themselves. No shift in consciousness is required and no additional attunements or initiations are necessary.

After my initial Reiki experiences, I embarked on a journey to integrate Reiki into my other healing modalities in my work and life. I took Second Degree Reiki within a few weeks. And when Third Degree Reiki was offered after Mrs. Hawayo Takata passed the Reiki keys to her successors, I became the tenth Reiki Master/Teacher in the West.

Reiki has been an integral part of my life and work since I first studied it. Second degree Reiki facilitates healing at a distance and transcends time and space dimensions as we consciously experience them. This workbook is designed for those who have studied Second Degree Reiki and who want to work on themselves at depth to clear past issues and/or to gain clarity about past experiences using Reiki healing energy to expand their consciousness.

The book is laid out primarily to record impressions from treatments. Based on my clinical experiences, the treatments result in profound clearings and transformations in those who use them.

I look forward to hearing from my readers about their experiences. You can contact me at ehp@nobleenergywellness.com.

In Loving Light,

Eleanor Haspel-Portner, Ph.D.

Eleanor Haspel-Portner, Ph.D.
Mount Pleasant, South Carolina

♦ ♦ ♦

INTRODUCTION

Mrs. Hawayo Takata passed Reiki, a tool for healing and wholeness, to us through her successors. With the study of First Degree Reiki, your hands became a channel for transmitting pure white light energy upon physical contact with living matter. The experience of First Degree Reiki generally has a profound effect on its students. With no alteration of consciousness through meditation, the healing energies of Reiki flow through the body on contact. No one needs any special attainment of supernatural or mystical powers to learn Reiki.

As a student of Reiki, upon receiving the First Degree that activates energy transmissions, you become a channel of the highest vibration energies known. As a channel of healing energies, with First Degree, you used Reiki on yourself and others to facilitate healing on whatever level was needed to achieve wholeness.

By its very nature, Reiki energy works naturally toward wholeness. Reiki energy is life force energy, and it moves in a spiraling formation much as the energy of creation moves in a spiral formation. This pattern of movement flows with life toward health consciousness, i.e., toward wholeness.

Through the years of my work with Reiki, many students expressed a deepening sense of inspiration and empowerment after being attuned to the different levels of Reiki. While each person experiences Reiki energy differently, most people genuinely feel something happening in their hands, on those that they touch, and within themselves. Reiki unlocks a white light healing power that already exists within each of us and, in illuminating that force, it connects us more cohesively to our life force energy. Taken from another perspective, people often feel a personal transformation.

As you become aware of yourself holding or channeling this Reiki healing light, you might experience subtle changes, while other people might experience dramatic transformations. After working with Reiki energy, you might feel drawn to practice Reiki and to continue with Second and sometimes Third Degree (Mastery), partly because it helps you better understand aspects of light and how you experience holding this light and this life force energy.

With Reiki, a deepening understanding that you are more, even than a holder of the light, grows within. You are a conduit and transmitter of light. The more you comprehend this, the more freedom you feel in all aspects of your life. Students often remark that they feel energized when they do Reiki on others. During Reiki, healing energy passes through you. This energy runs through everyone, joining everyone together as it heals you. No personal power is ever used in Reiki.

Second Degree Reiki allows you to move beyond the limits of physical space into another dimension of experience. The profound experience of First Degree Reiki becomes magnified and expands with the Second Degree Reiki, as it becomes activated through a set of energy transmissions. With Second Degree Reiki, you become a channel directing white light energy through time and space. Healing can be done at a distance on one or more individuals in the present, past, or future. With Second Degree Reiki, you might feel a stirring excitement as you did with First Degree Reiki — a sense that a deep knowing is being re-awakened within you.

When working with consciousness, you will likely experience a deep sense of recognition for those components that draw together unifying knowledge in its symbolic form. Reiki activates some of the recognition of the energetic components of this knowledge without your mind having to grasp information intellectually. All humans enter an energetic field of unity when they are asleep because, at that time, their consciousness shifts away from mental analysis and the interpretations it carries, and away from the field of human interaction. Thus, during sleep, you move beyond time and space.

The drive to regain full consciousness or full awareness is likely heightened in you through your experience of Reiki. In Second Degree Reiki classes, you learn how to do a Second Degree Reiki treatment on others and yourself. Most students of Reiki explore its usefulness; they do treatments regularly after learning the symbols and having the energy transmissions. Thus, the richness of Reiki has undoubtedly been revealed many times over.

Following a regular program when working on your unconscious level is essential for wholeness to manifest as it integrates fully with your psyche. When you begin to work on your "process," it usually serves you well to record your dreams so you can learn how to decode the symbolic messages in these dreams. Dreams can open doors into the collective unconscious because they are written by the higher mind, by the level of your archetypal connection to an awareness that extends beyond your conscious mind and emotions. In addition, information that emerges in a dream is most likely the primary process thinking that predates language, and how you "told yourself" a story about what you perceived, heard, felt, or knew. Thus, by accessing and working on that process in its non-verbal form, using Reiki, you can bypass the conscious mind and impact your psyche at the level that you experienced something. Thus, transformation is likely and possible in this state of consciousness.

The Self communicates with/to you in symbolic form because symbols carry a richness that transcends time, space, and words. The symbols of dreams often depict awareness that emerges from deep layers of your being and which, to the educated observer, occur cross-culturally and historically through the ages. Thus, a dream may carry an image that, when expanded, reveals an idea that another dreamer, in another time and place, also had. These images come out of the depths of your psyche; they have energy that often carries a great deal of power. Jung called such images archetypes and contrasted them to images that relate only to an individual's emotional life.

The Self exists in a deep level of your being. You know that your experience of who you are has remained relatively constant and familiar throughout your life. You have a sense of yourself in specific ways that remain stable despite changes in your outer life, e.g., changes in your environment, weight, appearance, and family situation. How well you relate your functional life to your more profound being, your Self, largely determines your level of consciousness or integrated wholeness. To the extent that you fully manifest and communicate with yourself, you manifest and radiate wholeness.

While in-depth analysis or deep self-reflection provides an essential tool for expanding into the Self, the further flowering of the spiritual meaning or connections of the Self may be facilitated by Reiki. Reiki activates centers of awareness that extend beyond the personal realm. Reiki taps into the archetypal levels of consciousness that allow you to reach beyond the limits of the mind and your physical being to experience the Self and the other energies.

A vital recognition begins in consciousness as you continue using Reiki. As the Reiki energy flows through you physically and emotionally, the channels clogged or muddied by personal experiences start to clear. As a result of clearing these channels, energies flow without resistance. The integration within and beyond you can then happen more quickly.

Just as analytic work expands when the spiritual meaning beyond the personal dimension enters the picture, Reiki work expands as one utilizes analytical tools to direct the cleansing process consciously.

What This Manual & Journal Covers

This Manual & Journal help Second Degree Reiki students utilize the profound energy of Reiki. When used directedly, you can clear problems in your life more rapidly. Combining useful analytic tools with the power of Reiki opens some inspiring doors into realms that are only now beginning to be explored and documented.

Since the wide dissemination of Reiki following Mrs. Takata's death in 1980, the exploration, development, and integration of Reiki into Western life and the Western psyche became the responsibility of Reiki Master/Teachers. The first task in Reiki always requires using Reiki on yourself to the fullest extent, allowing wholeness or integrative capacity to demonstrate how and what Reiki does.

You may need help structuring your internal relationship. Because your complexity goes beyond what your mind can comprehend, Reiki structure provides a focus that allows a safe journey inward into unknown spaces. As a Reiki student, you have a significant advantage over others since through practice, you experience profound levels of multidimensionality. You already possess keys to enlightenment. The discovery of the full power of the energies that Reiki unlocks requires focusing via treatments.

As a Second Degree Reiki student, you have undoubtedly done First Degree treatments on yourself and others. This Manual assumes that you have been initiated into Second Degree Reiki by a qualified Reiki Master/Teacher. See page page 47, How to Do a Second-Degree Reiki Treatment, to make sure you know the correct method of treatment for absent healing and that you have a level of comfort with the Second Degree Reiki symbols. If you have doubts about the Reiki Symbols, check with your teacher.

This Manual assumes that you treat yourself and others at a distance. It also assumes that you know how to treat more than one person at a time. Given these assumptions, the focus here will be to review all the Reiki Positions and what they treat and then structure some treatments that can facilitate clearing your personal issues and memories. You then have a clearer channel connecting your conscious and unconscious Self. During this pursuit, you will often work on others who have been significant to you. Healing will occur to both you and them during this process.

After a treatment, you reap significant benefits by writing down your feelings, images, and thoughts. By doing this, a channel of expression opens, making visible in concrete form what occurred psychically. As your unconscious moves into conscious awareness, and as you allow it to have tangible energy or form, you can more easily become unattached to the structure. You can examine or relate to the material and experience your relationship more explicitly.

Specific guidelines might be helpful in how you frame questions to yourself during and after treatment. These guidelines are based on ways of communicating with minimal interpretations of the images, so the depth of associations on the unconscious level of awareness finds expression in this most direct way. Many of these questions are based on the brilliant work of David Grove and Cei Davies Linn.

By recording your process during treatment, you will reconstruct many incidents of your life. A great deal of information may surface about yourself. New and unknown aspects of your Self-awareness will probably appear. Allow these energies to emerge. Allow the feelings and images. Allow thoughts, both positive and negative. Remain open, trusting,

A new you will begin to emerge. Further awareness will start to develop. Allow and enjoy this process. The journey through yourself contains more fascination than any other journey you ever will take. Commit time and energy to derive the fullest experience possible.

Contact your Reiki teacher or another qualified professional for guidance if you encounter any difficulties.

How to Use This Manual & Journal

This Manual & Journal offers a variety of ways to work with your process. No two people have the same style of approaching their psyche because no two people are exactly alike. Your discovery of your unique way of being and approach to your environment and life can emerge from your involvement and dedication to working with this Manual & Journal.

The book is divided into two primary sections for treating yourself. The first section approaches the process developmentally. The second section approaches the process structurally. Some people prefer to jump from section to section to experience and integrate both perspectives simultaneously as they progress. Others will feel more comfortable completing one section at a time in sequence before moving on to the next one. Other people may elect their unique approach. Allow yourself the freedom to find your style. No single path has been determined as the right path, and all systems, if followed to completion, end in integrated wholeness.

Developmental treatments focus on the natural unfolding process of the personality. In the course of life events, as well as interactions with significant people, reactions occur that cause one to feel specific ways. How progress through your life span has altered or directed you in particular practices rather than other ways shows your development. We all go through certain stages of this development process. Certain times in our lives make some feelings more vulnerable to change and alteration than others. In the developmental section, you will have an opportunity to look at yourself from the standpoint of significant influences on your growth that resulted in specific personality patterns. As you treat yourself with Second Degree Reiki throughout your life, you will find memories and feelings resurfacing. Continued work in these areas of your life will result in new emerging patterns of being.

Structural treatments focus on how parts of your being work together to achieve ultimate harmony. The components of your being exist before birth. These elements relate to each other in specific ways based on certain experiences and your concept of yourself and your life. How these parts exist functionally can be explored, assessed, and focused for wholeness.

The synthesis of these ways of viewing yourself comes together in relationships. Relationships refer to interactions between two or more entities. A relationship exists within you regarding how you interact with your consciousness internally, and relationships exist between you and others. Treatments in both realms will clarify and amplify your awareness of "who you are."

In addition, you will probably note that as you begin to work more intensively with your Self, dreams will emerge more vividly. Dreams will facilitate your journey through your Self if you record your dreams in the relevant section of this Manual & Journal. You can then expand your dreams for decoding using a combination of analytic tools with Reiki energies. This process promises to be exciting.

In all instances, using this book, you will be recording your observations when you do a treatment. Over time, patterns will begin to be visible to you with which you will become familiar. Roots, developmentally, or beliefs, structurally, will become clear. The pathways to your Self will become more explicitly accessible.

Enjoy your process.

THE REIKI TREATMENT AND HAND POSITIONS

Doing a First-Degree Reiki Treatment

Once you have gone through your Reiki Attunement and have active Reiki energy in your hands when you touch any living being, you are ready to do Reiki treatments on yourself and on other people, plants, and animals.

In order to do a Reiki treatment, you do not need any preparation and your state of mind is not relevant to the treatment. The pure white light energy of Reiki will flow from your hands upon touching a living being.

To prepare for a treatment, make sure you and whomever you are treating is in a comfortable setting and can remain undisturbed. The treatment takes about an hour. Before starting, wash your hands and make sure you are well-hydrated.

In a Reiki Treatment, there are four Head positions, five Front Positions, and five Back Position. In addition, there are a few additional hands-on positions specific to a man or a woman, highlighting areas where additional healing frequency energy is welcomed.

The positions in this manual are laid out for easy reference and include notes from my initial First Degree Reiki Class with Mrs.

Takata present in June, 1977. At the time of the class, I did not know anything about Reiki, but I knew that having Mrs. Takata at the class was important. Thus, during the class I took copious notes and learned some nuances that Mrs. Takata shared from her years of treating people using Reiki.

I have incorporated all my notes so they are easy to read and keep for quick reference, covering all the Reiki positions as well as some additional positions that are helpful to know and use.

When doing a treatment, the fingers are always together, and the hands are next to each other as in the diagrams illustrating each Reiki position. With First Degree Reiki, it is necessary to stay on each position for 5 minutes. At the end of the 5 minutes, move to the next position. Always treat using all the positions, and if there is an issue, e.g., knee pain, go to the that specific area after you finish all the other positions. The reason for this is that you want to treat the whole person and the source of the issue which may not have originated in the painful area.

It is also important to note that it is not necessary to physically touch the person you are working on. You can hold your hand slightly above the body and the energy will penetrate as though your hand is on the body. People are often aware of the energy flow.

You do not have to focus or concentrate during a treatment. Thus, you can do treatments on yourself when you are watching television, stopping at traffic lights, or even sitting in a classroom listening to a lecture. The main point is to use your Reiki healing hands as much and as often as you can to reap the most benefit.

Reiki Head Positions

The First Head Position has the following benefits in each of Field of Awareness

Rejuvenates your body through the pituitary gland, the master gland that balances hormones. Use this position when you want to clear your head and refocus in a relaxed way. This position is very important for diabetics.

MENTAL WORLD

Enhances clarity
Focuses thoughts
Focuses feelings
Relaxes your mind
Focuses concentration
Maximizes centering

SPIRITUAL WORLD

Activates the Sixth Chakra (The Third Eye Center).

Allows knowing and vision to expand into another dimension

Helps in meditation to open the Crown Center

First Head Position

**Position Hands Together,
Thumbs Toward Ears**

Dark Blue Represents the Ajna Chakra

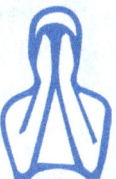

EMOTIONAL WORLD

Calms your mind
Turns your focus inward
Relaxes your mind and body
Shuts out external stimuli
Reduces overall stress

PHYSICAL WORLD

Balances the hypothalamus and pituitary glands

Helps:
Eyes, Sinus, Nose, and Allergy problems

Improves and helps heal:
Teeth, Upper Jaw, Ear Problems, Vertigo

Reiki Head Positions

The Second Head Position has the following benefits in each of Field of Awareness

Rejuvenates your body through balancing the hemispheres of the brain, resulting in clarity and focus of thoughts and relief from anxiety and stress. When your brain hemispheres are balanced, your calm, clear thinking is enhanced. Use this position when you have difficulty focusing and need clarity of mind.

MENTAL WORLD

Helps:
Balance your brain hemispheres
Enhance memory
Mental clarity
Clear depression
Increase alertness
Heighten creativity
Integrate thought

SPIRITUAL WORLD

Activates:
The Crown Chakra
Higher awareness
Expanded consciousness

Enhances:
Clarity of mind
Awareness
Psychic openness

Second Head Position

**Palms at Temples,
Fingers Together at Crown**

Purple Represents the Crown Chakra

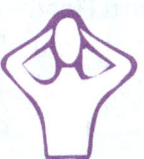

EMOTIONAL WORLD

Helps:
Relieve stress and worry
Calm anxiety
Decrease depression
Enhance dream recall
Centering
Focus your mind
Balance the hemispheres of your brain

PHYSICAL WORLD

Works on:
Pituitary and pineal glands (from lateral angle)

Helps:
Headaches
Dizziness
Shock
Motion sickness
Pain
TMJ

Facilitates the release of endorphins.

Reiki Head Positions

The Third Head Position has the following benefits in each of Field of Awareness

Rejuvenates and balances your body through the hypothalamus, the center of the brain that regulates the autonomous nervous system. This position helps with overall well-being and is especially helpful in falling asleep and in remembering dreams. It activates the cranial and vagus nerves.

MENTAL WORLD

Helps:
Balance your autonomic nervous system
Build your sense of well-being
Relaxed comfort
Reduce pain
Facilitate dream recall

SPIRITUAL WORLD

Balances mental well-being
Regulates the release of hypothalamic hormones

Enhances:
Clear expression of thoughts
Clear expression of ideas

Increases productivity

Expands multidimensional consciousness

Third Head Position

Fingers Together at Back of Head, Palms at Base of Head

Dark Blue Represents the Ajna Chakra

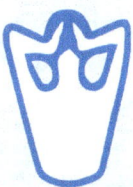

EMOTIONAL WORLD

Activates the back of your head to balance your third eye center for increased awareness

Enhances:
Perceptual awareness and receptivity of higher energies
Processing of higher energy frequencies
with increased ease and comfort

PHYSICAL WORLD

Works on hypothalamus:
Controls autonomic processes such as
blood presure, heartbeat, breathing

Helps:
Weight loss
Improve balance and coordination
Facilitate sleep induction
Relieve headaches

Reiki Head Positions

The Fourth Head Position has the following benefits in each of Field of Awareness

Rejuvenates your body through your thyroid and parathyroid glands, the master glands for balancing your metabolism and blood pressure. Since your Throat is the Power center for manifestation in the world, balancing this center enhances self-expression and self-esteem. Higher consciousness is enhanced in this position. If you have difficulty expressing yourself, energizing your throat may breakdown your fears and resistance to speaking. This position is important for lymphatic drainage.

MENTAL WORLD

Helps:
Balance your throat
Bring clarity of expression

Stabilizes:
The connection of your words with thoughts

Allows:
Your clarity to manifest

SPIRITUAL WORLD

Builds up:
Throat as a power for your center of communication and creative expression
Higher energies that gain expression through your throat, enhancing their manifestation

Fourth Head Position

Hands Around Throat

Light Blue Represents the Throat Chakra

EMOTIONAL WORLD

Balances:
Metabolism
Circulation

Helps:
Control anger   Enhance empowered feelings
Increase self-esteem   Enhance self-confidence

Facilitates:
Release of pent-up emotions

PHYSICAL WORLD

Helps:
Thyroid functioning   Throat issues
Parathyroid functioning   Tonsil, adenoid problems
Balance metabolism   Allergies
Regulate blood pressure   Bronchial problems

Activates:
Thymus gland and lymphatic system drainage

Reiki Front Positions

The First Front Position has the following benefits in each of Field of Awareness

Because this position works on your heart, lungs, and thymus gland, it opens you to your soul connection with the Divine. The more you experience this connection, the easier it becomes to recognize it in others. Reiki energy flows through the Heart Center in a frequency of Divine love and light. Balancing through a Reiki treatment opens you to experience the healing love of the Divine.

MENTAL WORLD

Helps:
Harmonious attitudes
Center thoughts and images
Brings you an integrative sense of clarity

SPIRITUAL WORLD

Opens your Heart Chakra to love
that transcends the personal level of your being

Connects you with the soul level of others
and with their higher selves

First Front Position

Hands at Level of Heart, Fingertips Touching

Green Represents the Heart Chakra

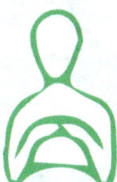

EMOTIONAL WORLD

Works on:
Heart center

Builds:
Trust
Courage
Positive self-esteem

Balances:
Anger
Negative feelings

Promotes:
Good feelings
Loving feelings

Reduces sadness

PHYSICAL WORLD

Works on:
Heart and lungs
Circulation
Thymus gland, positively affecting the immune system

Relieves:
Asthma
Chest wall pressure and pain

Reiki Front Positions

The Second Front Position has the following benefits in each of Field of Awareness

Realigns and balances your Solar Plexus Chakra including major organs of digestion and detoxification. When balanced, you are likely to experience more clarity and freedom from daily stressors. You are likely to experience more even emotional responses and less reactivity. When you have digestive issues, this position may be helpful.

MENTAL WORLD

Releases:
Power motive
Anger

Helps:
Mental clarity through centering
Cleansing your body of cloudy thoughts
related to bodily functions
Foster kindness

SPIRITUAL WORLD

Opens you to their your power
without the need for control

Respects your individual control or free choice

Facilitates your acceptance of the
ebb and flow of life energies

Second Front Position

Hand Under Breast, Fingertips Touching

Yellow Represents the Solar Plexus Chakra

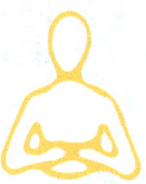

EMOTIONAL WORLD

Eases:
Fears   Negativity

Releases:
Stress generated by your body functions
Need to be in control of things

Promotes relaxation

PHYSICAL WORLD

Covers major organs:
Liver   Pancreas
Spleen Gall bladder
Stomach

Helps:
Digestion
Detoxification and processes of major body functions
Relieve digestive discomfort

Reiki Front Positions

The Third Front Position has the following benefits in each of Field of Awareness

Balances the Lower part of your Solar Plexus Chakra that includes your liver and the stomach. Digestive issues relax and release through treatments on this area. As your body releases tension in this area of your body, your mental fogginess and tiredness diminish.

MENTAL WORLD

Helps:
Clear your body of fogginess that interferes with mental clarity

Clears:
Depression
Confusion

SPIRITUAL WORLD

Your Solar Plexus Chakra helps:
Release your need for control or for acceptance
Keep your focus on the present moment
Release your past associations that hinder conscious living

Third Front Position

**Hands Just Above the Waist
Fingers Touching**

Yellow Represents the Solar Plexus Chakra

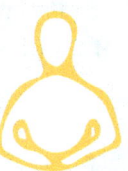

EMOTIONAL WORLD

Builds:
Self-confidence
Relaxation

Reduces Stress:
Releases your need for control or for acceptance
Facilitates your acceptance of self and others
Releases past associations that interfere with the present

PHYSICAL WORLD

Covers:
Lower part of your liver
Small and large intestines
Lower stomach

Relaxes and aids your digestion

Reduces pain from indigestion

Reiki Front Positions

The Fourth Front Position has the following benefits in each of Field of Awareness

Focused energy in your pelvis balances your sexual organs as well as your large and small intestines. When in equilibrium, your sense of adaptability and flexibility allow you to be creative and related to others. Your energy field becomes more powerful in attracting what you need. Sexual energy flows from this chakra. Use this position to help with menstrual cramps.

MENTAL WORLD

Increases:
Your Flexibility of thinking
Your adaptability

Releases:
Fear
Rigidity

SPIRITUAL WORLD

Focuses energy on:
Pelvic, Sexual Chakra

Opens you to the connections and relatedness of energy vibrations between living things
Magnetizes your energy field

Fourth Front Position

**Hands Below The Waist
Fingers Touching**

Orange Represents the Sex Chakra

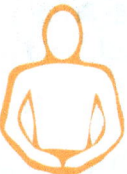

EMOTIONAL WORLD

Frees your sexual energy from conditioned patterns
Alleviates your fears and anxiety
Builds your confidence

PHYSICAL WORLD

Covers:
Pelvis
Ovaries and uterus
Prostate
Bladder
Large and small intestines

Helps:
Release toxins
Migraines associated with digestive imbalances
Constipation and diarrhea
Abdominal pain

Reiki Front Positions

The Fifth Front Position has the following benefits in each of Field of Awareness

The Root Chakra is the foundation from which you operate, it relates to your values and your strength, and it is the basis of your self-esteem and confidence. Circulation is enhanced in this position and thus, as Reiki energy moves through you, it clears any blockages and frees you up to take a stand that aligns with your core being.

MENTAL WORLD

Clarifies your assumptions that form the foundation of your thinking

Rids you of negative debris

SPIRITUAL WORLD

The Root Chakra anchors and supports your physical well-being

Important in clearing your body so your foundation is firm

Fifth Front Position

**Hands Over Groin
V-Shaped Fingers Touching**

Red Represents the Root Chakra

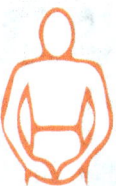

EMOTIONAL WORLD

Helps:
Build your confidence
Self-esteem

Clarifies values which are important to you
and that form the basis of your feelings

PHYSICAL WORLD

Covers:
Root position over groin

Builds:
Physical strength by generating energy through
the base of your trunk

Works on:
Genitals
Groin area
Circulation to your legs (leg lymphatics)

Reiki Back Positions

The First Back Position has the following benefits in each of Field of Awareness

Relaxation and release from your neck and throat allow energy to move more freely through your body reducing inflammation and pain and connecting mind and body in ways that enhance your overall well-being and communication. Sitting with your hand on your neck in this position can be very freeing and relaxing. Use it often.

MENTAL WORLD

Works on:
Relaxation
Centering
Clarity of expression
Collects your thoughts for mental stability

SPIRITUAL WORLD

Balances:
Throat Chakra
The nervous system

Overall:
Connects your mind and body
Sense of your integration of being
All communication is enhanced

First Back Position

Between Upper Shoulders,
Below Neck Hands Form a V-Shape
Light Blue Represents the Throat Chakra

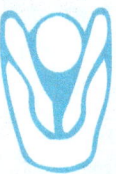

EMOTIONAL WORLD

Facilitates:
Tension release
Stress reduction
Control of anger
Increase in your self esteem

Release of pent up emotion resulting in:
Positive feelings
Self-confidence
Freedom of your mind to deal with feelings

PHYSICAL WORLD

Relaxes:
Neck and trapezius
Upper lungs
Upper spinal cord (C7-T4)

Reduces pain and inflammation
from tight muscles and joints

Reiki Back Positions

The Second Back Position has the following benefits in each of Field of Awareness

Relaxed breathing from the enhanced energy of Reiki allows your heart to open and your circulatory system to flow. When you feel that your thoughts can flow freely, you are likely to feel empowered and clear. Note: This is a difficult position to do on yourself. To make it easier use one hand at a time. Because it activates the lungs it is an important position to work at.

MENTAL WORLD

Clears your mind by freeing your body of impurities in your circulatory system

Helps you feel like thoughts can travel through the air

SPIRITUAL WORLD

Activates:
Your Heart Chakra

Lets you open to the energy around and to respond with a clear sense of yourself

Second Back Position

Hand on Lower Shoulder Next to Spine

Green Represents The Heart Chakra

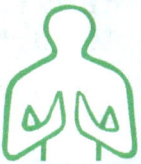

EMOTIONAL WORLD

Relaxes tension almost immediately.

Lets you catch your breath
so you can handle whatever is before you

Helps:
Center and calm your emotions
Build courage

PHYSICAL WORLD

Helps:
Lungs, heart, circulation
Energy in your body
Breathing

Your left shoulder relaxes:
Your body
Your nervous system

Your right shoulder helps:
Gall bladder
Enhances sleep
Heart and lung conditions

Reiki Back Positions

The Third Back Position has the following benefits in each of Field of Awareness

Energy flows into your kidney and adrenal glands, helping manage stress and relieving any confusion, fears, and toxicity in your body. This position is easy to do on yourself when you are waiting in lines. Trust is enhanced in this position as is the impulse toward action. By working on this position extra, you build more adrenal resilience.

MENTAL WORLD

Helps clear your mind by relieving it of:
Confusion
Extraneous thoughts, fears, angst

Enhances:
Clarity
Logic

SPIRITUAL WORLD

Builds a sense of ability to:
Take action
Accomplish things

Helps you feel:
Trusting and confident
In touch with higher energies
In touch with your purposes

Third Back Position

**Small of Back
Fingers Touching**

Yellow Represents the Solar Plexus Chakra

EMOTIONAL WORLD

Relieves stress
Releases fear

Helps you feel:
Secure
Trusting

Balances your emotions

PHYSICAL WORLD

Helps:
Kidneys and adrenal glands   Immune system
Pancreas and liver   Shock and whiplash

Gives you increased stamina

Very important position for:
Clearing your body of toxins
Handling stress

Reiki Back Positions

The Fourth Back Position has the following benefits in each of Field of Awareness

Security and trust gain energy from activating this chakra and its meridians. Balancing your nervous system enhances your immune system and builds clarity and life force energy. This position is near the "Gate of Life" a key area in the back where the energy moves up your body. Energy in this area of the back is important for opening your consciousness.

MENTAL WORLD

Helps clear your mind by relieving it of:
Confusion
Extraneous thoughts

Enhances:
Clarity
Logic

SPIRITUAL WORLD

Works on:
Solar Plexus Chakra
Generating primal energy

Used As:
Life force energy
Energy that forms as the foundation of all action

Fourth Back Position

Base of spine forming V
Orange Represents the Sex Chakra

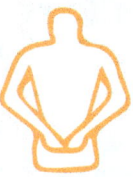

EMOTIONAL WORLD

Opens you to your own base of energy

Generates:
Security
Trust and integrity

From this point emerges greater energy

PHYSICAL WORLD

Base of your spine, coccyx

Helps your nervous system:
Balance energy
Generate chi energy

Energizes and builds:
Sexual function
Stamina

Reiki Back Positions

The Fifth Back Position has the following benefits in each of Field of Awareness

Comfort and security become more stable, and you are energized to keep grounded when Reiki activates the Root Chakra. Security comes from your inner confidence that you are balanced and calm. Using this position strengthens your ability to stand your ground.

MENTAL WORLD

Calms your mind
Calm and soothing energy

Gives:
Confidence
Ease to thinking

SPIRITUAL WORLD

Works:
Through your Root Chakra

Enhances:
Your grounding process
Security of being

Balances your physical body

Fifth Back Position

On Buttocks

Red Represents the Root Chakra

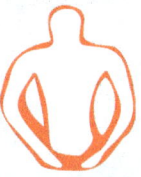

EMOTIONAL WORLD

Low key enhancement of:
Security
Confidence

Not an action oriented position

PHYSICAL WORLD

Works on:
The buttocks

Promotes:
Sense of comfort   Sense of security

Helps:
Warm your body   Relaxation and sleep

Good for:
Stroke   Bedridden
Sciatica

How to Do a Second Degree Reiki Treatment

A Second Degree Reiki Treatment can be done on an individual or on any number of individuals in a group. The use of Reiki Symbols in their proper form activates an energy transfer beyond the boundaries of time and space. It allows work at a distance, known as an "absent healing treatment."

There are three Reiki Symbols used in a Second Degree Reiki Treatment.

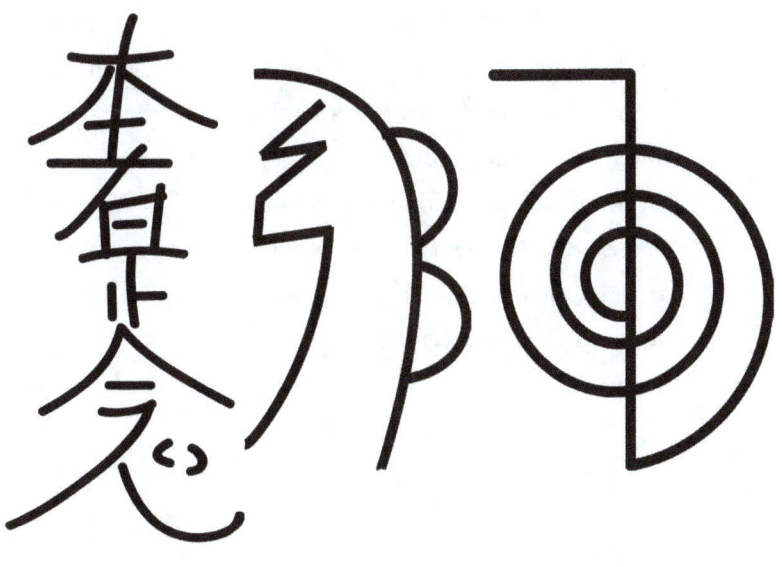

Hon Sha Ze Sho Nen   Sei He Ki   Cho Ku Rei

Illustration 1: All three Second Degree Reiki symbols

Hon Sha Ze Sho Nen sets up the intention for the treatment at a distance on a particular individual or group of individuals, i.e., on any living thing.

Sei He Ki accesses the unconscious layers of the target.

Cho Ku Rei sets the energy in motion directing it toward its target.

The treatment always follows the specific format and sequence of steps as outlined along with the symbols and how they are drawn and shown:

1. Identify the subject of your treatment.

2. Prepare yourself to receive the Reiki energy and to initiate your treatment.

3. Sit comfortably.

4. Draw: **Hon Sha Ze Sho Nen** once and say the words **Hon Sha Ze Sho Nen** three times as you imagine the symbol being drawn on the person's forehead. While you are stroking/drawing this symbol, know that your intention is healing for the highest good of the person on whom you are initiating the absent healing. The Hon Sha Ze Sho Nen sets up the absent treatment intent and accesses the energy field of the person on whom you are about to work to receive the treatment.

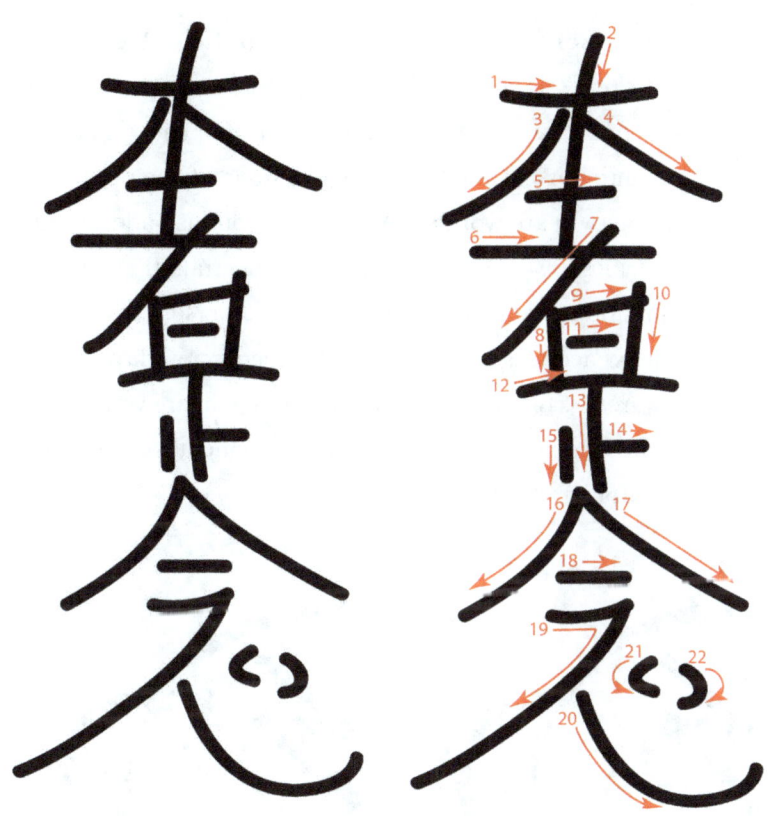

Illustration 2: Hon Sha Ze Sho Nen – Shown with and without stroking

5. Draw: **Sei He Ki** *once* and say the words **Sei He Ki** *three* times as you imagine this symbol on the person's forehead. As you stroke/draw this symbol know that your intention is healing for the highest good of the person on whom you are working. At this time you may address any specifics for the person, always being certain that you do not impose your wishes or will on that person. The Sei He Ki accesses and works on the unconscious layer of awareness of the individual on whom you are working. Thus, it alleviates psychological components of the issue or problem for healing.

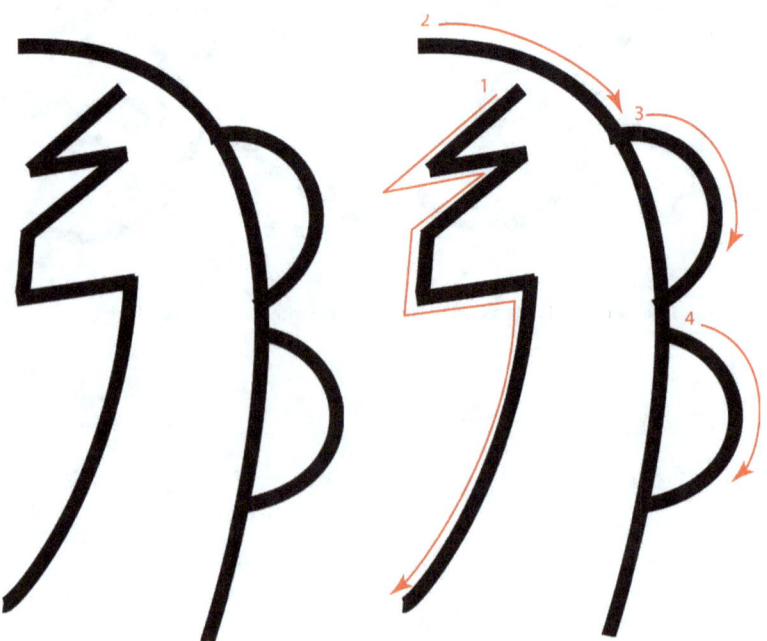

Illustration 3: Sei He Ki – Shown with and without stroking

6. Draw: **Cho Ku Rei** *once* and say the words **Cho Ku Rei** *three* times as you imagine this symbol being drawn on the person's forehead. As you stroke/draw this symbol know that your intention is healing for the highest good for the person on whom you are working. The Cho Ku Rei activates and puts the healing energy in motion directing it to the person identified.

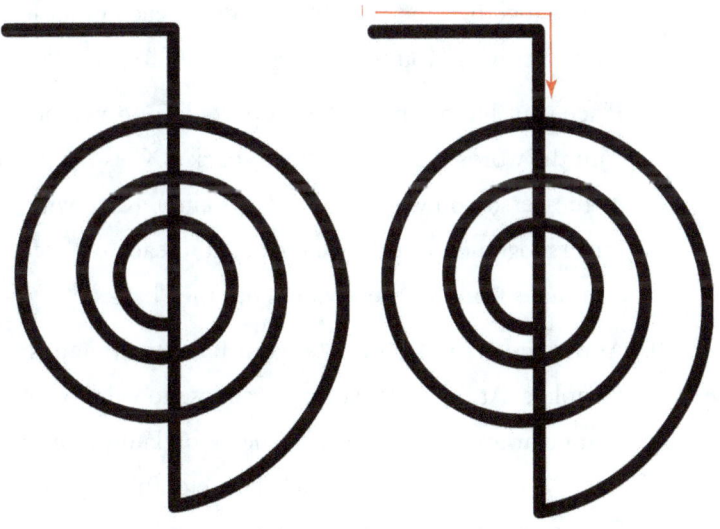

Illustration 4: Cho Ku Rei – Shown with and without stroking

7. Place your hands on a part of your own body with the words: Let this be "X's" head ("X" is the name of the person on whom you are working). Keep your fingers together and your hands next to each other for 5 minutes while you send energy to the "head."

8. Place your hands on a different part of your own body with the words: Let this be "X's" front ("X" is the name of the person on whom you are working). Keep your fingers together and your hands next to each other for 5 minutes while you send energy to the "front."

9. Place your hands on a different part of your own body with the words: Let this be "X's" back ("X" is the name of the person on whom you are working). Keep your fingers together and your hands next to each other for 5 minutes while you send energy to the "back."

10. At the end of the 15 minutes your basic treatment is complete. At this time, you may choose to work on a particular area of the person where you know a problem exists, e.g., a headache or backache, etc. In this case, you follow the same procedure, placing your hands on a different part of your own body with the words: Let this be "X's" *name the body part* ("X" is the name of the person on whom you are working). Continue working until you sense a change in the energy flow. You can work as long and on as many areas of the person or situation as you feel warranted.

11. Remove your hands from the sending mode and express appreciation to the person on whom you worked as well as to the higher forces for their help.

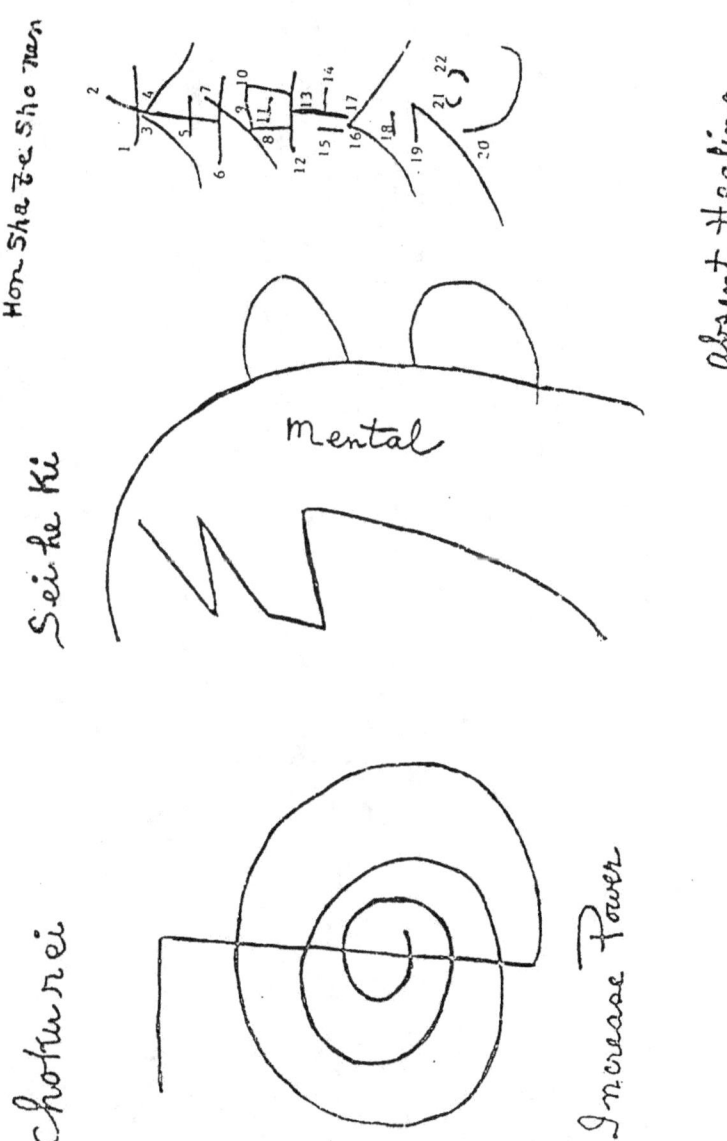

Illustration 5: Mrs. Takata's drawing of Second Degree Reiki symbols

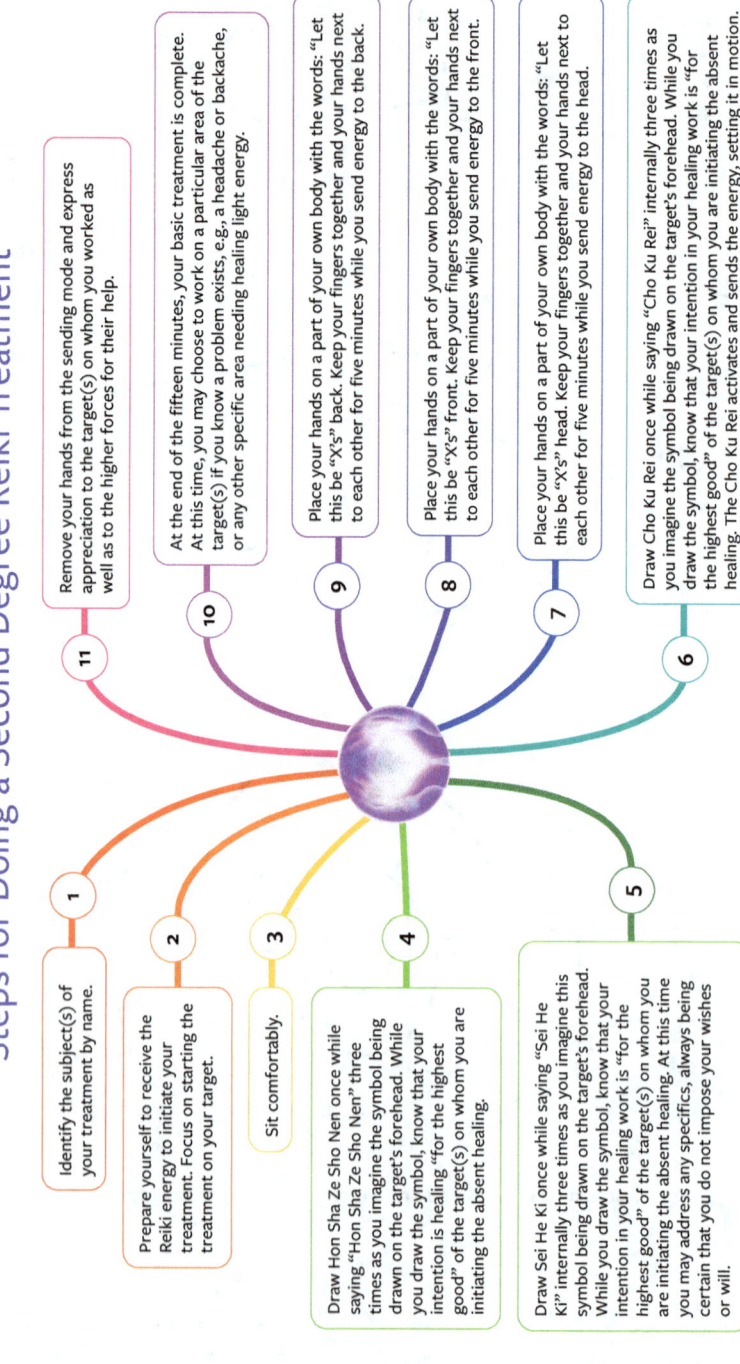

Developmental Treatments

Few of us can spontaneously remember our conception or birth, yet it represents highly significant markers for us psychologically, spiritually, physically, and mentally. Extensive Reiki work on your conception, gestation, and birth can lead to surprising and beneficial awareness. Be patient with these treatments. Do not rush. The time will prove to be well spent in the long run. Use this Manual & Journal to record your observations after you complete your treatment.

Treat your Self at the moment of your conception:

Treat your Self and your parents at your moment of conception:

Treat your Self during each month of your gestation. First Month:

Second Month:

Third Month:

Fourth Month:

Fifth Month:

Sixth Month:

Seventh Month:

Eighth Month:

Ninth Month:

Do additional treatments on your Self if you know of or sense any problems during your gestation. Treat repeatedly until the energies clear, i.e., flow freely and without your sensing the blockages.

Treat your Self and your mother during your gestation. At conception:

First Month:

Second Month:

Third Month:

Fourth Month:

Fifth Month:

Sixth Month:

Seventh Month:

Eighth Month:

Ninth Month:

Any issues or problems that you sense during this time require additional treatments.

Treat your parent's relationship during your gestation.
At conception:

First Month:

Second Month:

Third Month:

Fourth Month:

Fifth Month:

Sixth Month:

Seventh Month:

Eighth Month:

Ninth Month:

Treat your Self and your mother as labor began:

Treat your Self and your mother during labor:

Treat your Self during your birth:

Treat your mother during your birth:

Treat both your Self and your mother during your birth:

Note: During your growth, certain periods of development carry particular vulnerabilities. The following times represent such periods. Do treatments on your Self and on your family to access and to heal any disturbances during these times.

Treat your Self at six weeks of age:

Treat your Self and your family when you were six weeks old:

Treat your Self at three months of age:

Treat your Self and your family when you were three months old:

Treat your Self at six months of age:

Treat your Self and your family when you were six months old:

Treat your Self at eight months of age:

Treat your Self and your family when you were eight months old:

Treat your Self at ten months of age:

Treat your Self and your family when you were ten months old:

Treat your Self at one year of age:

Treat your Self and your family when you were one year old:

Treat your Self at eighteen months of age:

Treat your Self and your family when you were eighteen months old:

Treat your Self at two years of age:

Treat your Self and your family when you were two years old:

Treat your Self at two and a half years of age:

Treat your Self and your family when you were two and a half years old:

Note: These following treatments include significant periods of your development. For example, the time you learned to smile, got teeth, experienced fear of strangers, began to sit, walk, got separated from your mother, first talked, and used the toilet.
If these times have not surfaced, focus on doing treatments specifically at that time, e.g., treat "the time I said my first word," "the time I felt fear of a stranger," etc.

The birth of a sibling often represents a significant event in an individual's life. Such an event may require repeated treatments to access the importance of the event and the information that clears it of its unconscious components.

If you have a younger sibling do a treatment on your Self at the time your sibling came into your life.

Treat your Self and your sibling together:

Treat your Self on your first day of school:

Treat your Self and your first real friend:

Treat your Self at age five:

Treat your Self and your family when you were five years old:

Treat your Self when you learned to read:

Treat your Self and your favorite grade school teacher:

Treat your Self each year. Age 7:

Age 8:

Age 9:

Age 10:

Age 11:

Treat your Self as you entered puberty:

Treat your Self and your family as you entered puberty:

(Women) Treat your Self at your first menstruation:

Treat your Self when you learned your favorite sport:

Treat your Self on your first date:

Treat your Self and your family when you had your first date:

Treat your Self when you graduated from elementary school:

Treat your Self when you graduated from Junior High School:

Treat your Self when you graduated from High School:

Treat your Self when you got your driver's license:

Treat your Self when you learned to drive:

Treat your Self when you decided what to do when you graduated from High School:

Treat your Self at your first sexually charged party:

Treat your Self at the time of your first sexual experience:

Treat your Self and the person with whom you shared your first sexual experience:

Note: As life develops, one always confronts unexpected events that may have a profound effect on one's life. Some of these significant events may be:

Family occasions, yours and those in your family, e.g., marriages, birthdays, graduations:

Changes in school:

Moving from one home to another:

Divorce of parents or other relatives:

Deaths of any significant people in your life:

Getting a pet:

The death of a pet:

Important trips or memories:

Accidents:

Illnesses:

Visits to the Doctor:

Note: Explore some of these events or others that may be important for you and their effects on you. Generally, treating yourself, the other people involved, and the situation is wise. Paths diverge significantly when an individual enters adulthood. Nevertheless, specific developmental sequences emerge throughout the lifespan. Although many events may have affected you significantly, you will be able to see how to proceed from the following examples of treatments.

Treating Yourself Structurally

In order for you to feel whole, you must function in a harmonious way. When any part of you moves out of sync or out of alignment, you are likely to feel the shift and must adapt or compensate in some manner to accommodate it. Esoteric literature generally describes your body as functioning in four interrelated worlds often described as four interrelated bodies that work together as an integrated unified whole. These bodies are:

Your Physical Body - This body corresponds to your experienced physical body. Your physical body exists and interacts with the objective physical world of life and/or reality. In addition, your cells, your physiology, your brain, and your movements all function on this physical level, often without conscious intervention on your part. Think about the automatic way your body digests food, functions when you sleep, or "knows what to do" when you walk or move.

Your Spiritual Body - This body refers to your energy experience of connectedness between cosmic forces of the universe and how you manifest this energy in the physical world. Through this spiritual (or etheric) world all life connects. A full experience of your spiritual body allows you to experience the interconnectedness of all life and its unity. The kind of kinship you feel with those you love, the unity of human compassion that draws and drives you forward toward something greater than yourself constitutes the spiritual body. It is often experienced as an inner Knowing. I call it Knowing with a "K".

Your Emotional Body - This body carries your feelings that convey positive or negative charges of energy. Your issues deriving from personal experiences may become fixed in your emotional (or astral) body. Distress may arise because emotional reactions are often based in desires rather than in factual analysis of situations and may not align congruently with the higher Self or life purpose. Language mediates this layer of awareness because it codes non-verbal thought into form. When reality does not support what is coded from the past, disharmony results. It is this misalignment that causes discomfort; Reiki re-aligns the emotional body congruently to the higher Self, i.e., to the Spiritual Body.

Your Mental Body - This body carries thought patterns, interconnections, and associations based on analysis and understanding of the outer world. The component elements of consciousness get carried and integrated into the physical world through your mind. This body operates in the reality of your life interactions, making you vulnerable to environmental circumstances and how they affect your thinking. Taking dominion over this energy body is essential to balance because through it you have the power within your own mind to change thought patterns and belief systems that influence interactions in your life.

These four energy bodies function together as a whole. Awareness of Self as a whole and consciousness of various energy bodies can be helpful in pinpointing areas of particular strength or areas in you that lack clarity. When the four energy bodies work as an integrated whole, you feel life energy flowing smoothly—you feel a sense of well-being, i.e. happiness and health. Any disturbance in a particular "body" creates a sense of disturbance through your whole being. Go to www.nobleenergywellness.com for more information on how these bodies function in you. See the Mandala Illustration to see how all systems of esoteric knowledge integrate in a unified system.

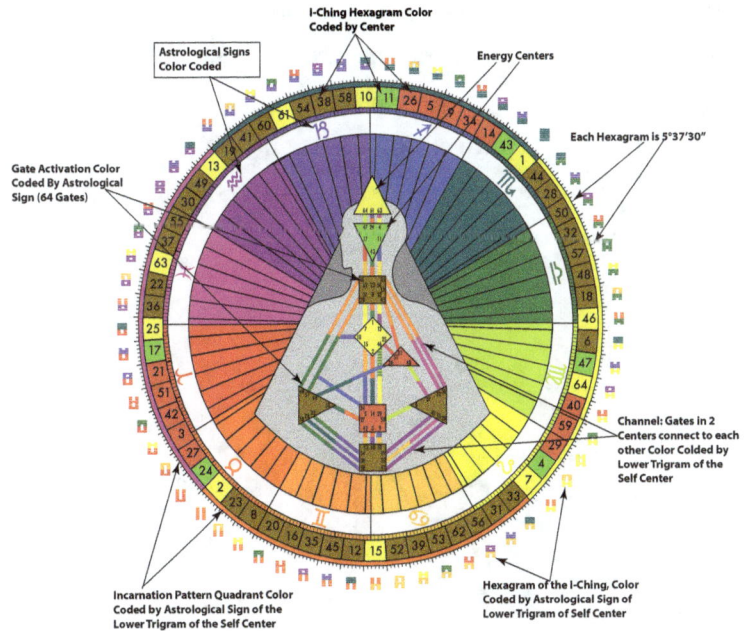

Illustration 6: Annotated 64-Gate Mandala used in Noble Energy Maps™
https://www.nobleenergywellness.com/mandala-of-synthesis/

With Second Degree Reiki you can harmonize your energetic bodies in an integrated way so you function optimally. Reiki energies touch all levels simultaneously, allowing you to expand your awareness of the structural elements involved in your functioning. This aspect of awareness will become more evident to you as you do some of the treatments in this section of the Manual & Journal.

Another way of thinking about and of organizing awareness about yourself is to describe the objective vs. the subjective areas of your life. This way of thinking may be used in to accomplish an understanding of how you organize resources in your Self to manifest in the world. Several treatments tap into this dimension.

Chakras have been described as energy centers in the body. In the Hindu Chakra System, seven major chakras have been described: the base/root chakra, the sexual/sensational chakra, the solar plexus chakra, the heart chakra, the throat chakra, the third eye chakra, and the crown chakra (Illustration 7). Each chakra centers in a different part of your body and relates to different aspects of your evolving consciousness.

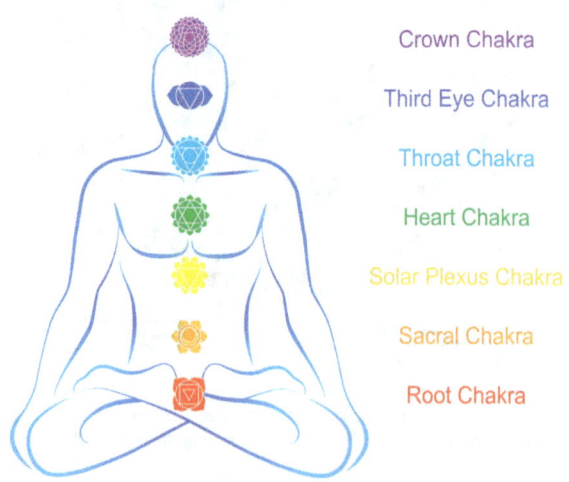

Illustration 7: The Hindu Chakra System

In the Kabalistic Tree of Life, energy centers are called Sephiroth. In the Tree of Life (Illustration 8), there are ten designated energy centers that connect through thirty-two paths of intelligence describing the process of evolving consciousness. As each task or path is completed in each of the four energy bodies, or worlds, as they are called in the Tree of Life, new awareness and discernment of subtleties of functioning become active.

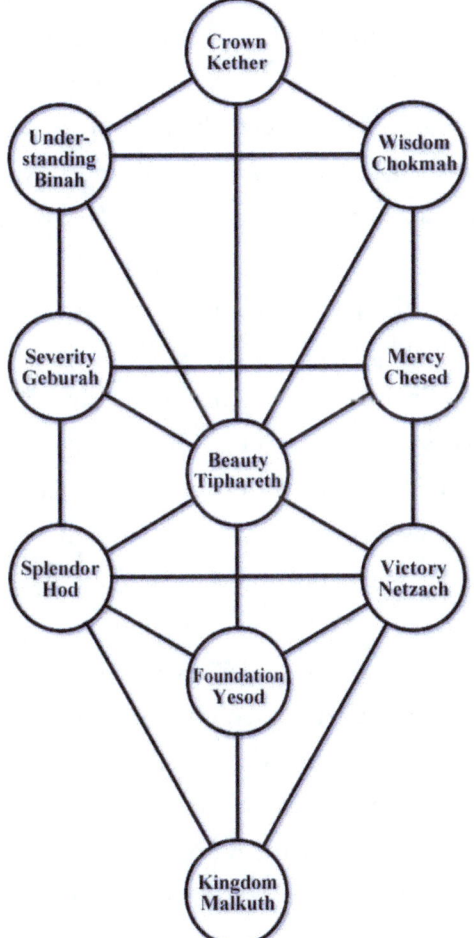

Illustration 8: The Tree of Life

As you explore your chakras and/or Sephiroth (paths of intelligence) using Second Degree Reiki you will be amazed, I am sure, to learn that your awareness and feelings mirror those of sages through the ages. You will tap into archetypal (collective group) levels of awareness in a very direct way. The experience of these dimensions will open you in unexpected ways.

Another structural dimension of your personality may be tapped by delving into what C.G. Jung described as your psychological type. Your "psychological type" describes the main way you process and organize information about the world and about your Self. Jung described four functions that encompass ways of perceiving or judging information about the world. He also described two primary attitudinal modes of organizing these functions.

The four functions and their organization in your personality determine your psychological type. Thus, you may be either predominantly an extrovert or predominantly an introvert. An extrovert directs their energy outward from the Self toward the objective world. If you are an extrovert your elationships in the world show in how you express your Self. An introvert dirests their energy of the Self inwardly toward their subjective world; if you are an introvert, your relationship with your inner world determines your self-experience. Within the framework of these two primary attitude modes of organizing energy, you have a dominant function type. The functions are: intuition, sensation, thinking, and feeling.

Expansion of these Types and an actual energy description of how you function may be learned from my work. I developed and scientifically document my work through **Noble Energy Maps™**, using multidimensional tools that describe Five Ways of Being (Types) and their functioning (www.nobleenergywellness.com). Studying this information lets you learn a great deal about your communication patterns and the perceptive or judging filters you impose upon the world and others. In addition, when you treat your "functional typology," you will begin developing those functions that you generally relegate to a secondary position within your Self. In Noble Energy Maps™, there are five Types defined. These types have been scientifically documented on 45,000 cases.

Noble Energy Maps™ describes the five types: Manifestor, Generator, Manifesting Generator, Projector, and Reflector. These Types correspond to Jungian types with the Manifesting Generator serving as an integrative type. The Manifesting Generator uses more than one strategy in functioning. The Manifestor is the Thinking type, the Generator is the Feeling type, the Projector is the Sensation type, and the Reflector is the Intuitive type.

You are about 95% likely to become a Manifesting Generator, i.e., someone who can make things happen when unconscious and conscious intention align and come to fruition in the world of form, when you live in your integrated auric energy field. (Research done by Eleanor Haspel-Portner, Ph.D. through Noble Sciences, LLC.) Thus, you are more than just your conscious and unconscious worlds that define waking consciousness. In addition, Noble Sciences provides you with an actual body energy map from which you can see your mechanical (genetic) structure. By working with Reiki on your actual body energy map. Get a copy of your energy map by emailing me at ehp@noblesciences.com with your birth date, time, and place of birth. You can bring about great awareness and change bypassing personality issues.

By doing the treatments on your attitude mode and functioning typology, you may learn a great deal about how these aspects work. Record your awareness before reading the explanatory sections in the Manual & Journal. You can then discover by self-reflection, and through intensive Reiki treatments, that you have the wisdom of other seekers. You will recognize how wise you really are.

Treat your Physical body:

Treat your Spiritual (Etheric) body:

Treat your Emotional (Astral) body:

Treat your Mental body:

Treat your Physical and Spiritual bodies:

Treat your Physical and Emotional bodies:

Treat your Physical and Mental bodies:

Treat your Spiritual and Emotional bodies:

Treat your Spiritual and Mental bodies:

Treat your Emotional and Mental bodies:

Treat your Physical, Spiritual, and Emotional bodies:

Treat your Spiritual, Emotional, and Mental bodies:

Treat your Physical, Spiritual, Emotional, and Mental bodies:

Treat your Objective Self:

Treat your Subjective Self:

Treat the relationship between your Objective and Subjective Selves:

Treat your Outer Self:

Treat your Inner Self:

Treat the relationship between your Outer and Inner Selves:

Question to ask: What differences or similarities have you noted in the treatments on the Objective-Subjective dimension as compared to the Outer-Inner dimension? [Notice in looking at this if you are different when you are alone vs. when you are with other people].

Treat your Extroverted Self (How you are when you are with other people in interactive settings):

Treat your Introverted Self (How you are internally and how you take things in):

Treat the relationship between your Extroverted and Introverted Self (How you balance your outer persona with your inner life):

Treat your Intuitive Self (How you know things):

Treat your Sensation Self (What you recognize about yourself):

Treat your Thinking Self (Manifestor Type/Mental Layer):

Treat your Feeling Self (How you respond to things internally):

Treat your Extroverted - Intuitive Self (How you bring your inner knowing into outer form):

Treat your Extroverted - Sensation Self (How you experience the world around you):

Treat your Extroverted - Thinking (How you orient yourself toward your world):

Treat your Extroverted - Feeling Self (How you respond and feel in the context of your daily life):

Treat your Introverted-Intuitive Self (How you know things and feel inwardly):

Treat your Introverted-Sensation Self (How you process information physically):

Treat your Introverted-Thinking Self (The stories you tell yourself about your life in an ongoing way):

Treat your Introverted-Feeling Self (How you feel about your life in an ongoing way):

Note: Qualities and characteristics that seem to be strongest in these treatments give clues to your inner process. Which psychological type do you believe you are based on your treatments?

Treat your Public Self:

Treat your Private Self:

Treat the relationship between your Public and Private Self:

Note: To treat a chakra, set up the image of treating your Self through that particular chakra. Then, do your symbols and treat the head, the front, and the back through that chakra system

Treat your Self through the Root Chakra:

Treat your Self through the Sexual Chakra:

Treat your Self through the Solar Plexus Chakra:

Treat your Self through the Heart Chakra:

Treat your Self through the Throat Chakra:

Treat your Self through the Third Eye Chakra:

Treat your Self through the Crown Chakra:

Treat the relationship between your Root Chakra and your Physical body:

Treat the relationship between your Sexual Chakra and your Emotional body:

Treat the relationship between your Solar Plexus chakra and your Mental body:

Treat the relationship between your Heart Chakra and your Spiritual body (Higher consciousness):

Treat the relationship between your Throat Chakra and your Spiritual body (transcendental awareness):

Treat the relationship between your Third Eye Chakra and your spiritual awakening:

Treat the relationship between your Crown Chakra and universal consciousness (light):

Hint: In doing the treatments on your Self structurally, a great deal of information will undoubtedly become available to you. At this point, you may find it useful to review the work you have done so far in your Manual & Journal. In order to review the material in a way that allows you continuity, choose a time to go over your writings when you will be relaxed and without time pressures. Begin reading and take notes. Write down or draw some representation of any significant patterns that begin to emerge (become clear to you). Note any paradoxes that you had to deal with or integrate in the course of your development or in order to function in the world. Begin to appreciate the high level of integrity along with the intelligence you manifested in your life when you learned the lessons you needed to learn. The evolution of your awareness always follows what you were ready to know and perceive. Make sure you express gratitude to your highest self for your developing awareness, and be certain to include a "because" statement with the gratitude that notes a tangible and concrete way you took authority to activate the gratitude.

Focus on areas that claimed extra energy positively or negatively for additional Reiki treatments.

♦ ♦ ♦

DREAMS

Throughout recorded history, dreams have played a significant role because they reveal what is unseen and unknown to man's conscious mind. However, understanding some of the ways in which dreams communicate did not take conscious shape until Freud's publication of the *Interpretation of Dreams*, first published in German in 1900. Science now accepts dreaming as a natural and necessary part of sleep. In fact, if you are interrupted during your dream cycle or cannot sleep for any extended period of time, your health will suffer.

You dream even when you don't recall the content of your dreams when awake. With some practice, however, you may find that you remember some of your dreams and can record them without too much difficulty. Your may ask, "what do my dreams mean, if anything, and what purpose do they serve?"

In the work of Noble Sciences, I documented that during sleep humans move into a different structural matrix of energy that allows communication with the collective symbolic (archetypal) layer of consciousness directly. This layer of awareness connects you to other living beings (spiritual dimension of consciousness, i.e., the spiritual world) and puts you in touch with things of which you are not consciously aware. During dreams, all parts or layers of your auric energy field, the Physical, Mental, Emotional, and Spiritual integrate.

Although everything connects with your deep self when you sleep, only some parts of the information are transferred to the waking part of your brain. The residues of symbolic information from dreams become accessible to you when you wake up. At that time, it is translated into a form you only partially perceive. Dreams that you remember cross over from one state of consciousness to another; it is this cross-over between layers of consciousness that makes dreams so difficult to recall in their fullest form.

Because dreams speak in symbolic form during sleep, when you try to describe dreams in words something gets lost in translation. Noble Sciences documents the way dream transitions happen. It also shows how you function in an integrated way all day, how your subconscious aligns and works, and your process by which intentions become manifested reality.

You are likely to find answers to many questions you have about your life and consciousness when you work with and use this Manual & Journal. Record your dreams in sequence with the date of their occurrence. Record any significant events that might be going on in your life at the time or within a week of the day you record your dream. When you feel ready to work on your dream to decode it, set aside some time. The following procedure can be used as a general guide in working with your dreams.

1. Read your dream through from beginning to end.
2. Treat your Self as the Dreamer and your Self as the Knower using Second Degree Reiki.
3. Write down each important image from the dream along with your associations to that image.
4. Treat each image that carries a strong energy for you with Second Degree Reiki.
5. Any figures that appear in the dream can be treated with Reiki. Write down associations about who they are or whom they remind you of.

As you can see, working with a dream will be time consuming. Take the time. Your dreams contain secrets of the cosmos, life, and awareness; dreams can reveal great wisdom. As you become comfortable with your dreams, you will begin to discover that inner figures relate to you repeatedly. Guiding figures of conscious understanding speak to you through your dreams.

As you become familiar with a dream figure you may want to expand your communication with that figure. You can do a treatment on the figure and on your Self (either a joint treatment or two separate treatments) and then you use "clean language" in delving deeper into the symbolic representations of the dream. Using "clean language" will allow you to trace the metaphoric coding of the symbol as it connects the worlds. Begin to delve into yourself by asking: "And what do I know about _____ now?" You can learn more about "clean language" by going to: http://www.nobleenergywellness.com. Deep awareness often emerges from working this way. Over time, you will find that certain inner figures and images become very important to you.

Through the use of **NobleEnergy Wellness**™, in conjunction with basic, as well as advanced Reiki levels, you have the tools needed to shift your life in profoundly transformational ways. Use these tools daily to increase self-discovery. Enjoy your process and have fun!

About the Author

Eleanor Haspel-Portner, Ph.D.

Eleanor Haspel-Portner, Ph.D. became involved in meditation and energy work in the early 1970's. Reiki came to her attention in 1977 when she enrolled in a Reiki class to determine if it had any validity. Mrs. Takata was present at the first degree Reiki class that Eleanor attended. After the first attunement Eleanor was instructed to go home that night and work on herself using the four Reiki head positions. She followed the instructions and when she awoke the next morning she noted that she could see without her glasses, which she wears for very severe myopia.

Something extraordinary had happened. Eleanor took this experience to mean that indeed there was validity to Reiki. After receiving the second Reiki attunement, Eleanor noted that her perfect vision lasted for an even longer period of time. She received all first-degree Reiki initiations and went on to study second degree Reiki. At that time Mrs. Takata did not make third degree Reiki available. Mrs. Takata passed the Reiki keys to others before her death in 1980; after she died Reiki became more generally available; Eleanor studied third degree Reiki in 1981. Eleanor is a long standing member of the Reiki Alliance.

Eleanor received her Ph.D. from The University of Chicago, Department on Comparative Human Development, one of the first interdisciplinary departments in the United States. Eleanor uniquely integrates her background and training in the Social Sciences (psychology, biology, anthropology, sociology) with esoteric studies. By applying multidimensional tools in **Noble Energy Welness and Noble Energy Maps**™ that she developed and validated, Eleanor helps people transform their lives. In private practice work as a clinical psychologist and coach since 1974, Eleanor helped thousands of individuals, couples, and groups synthesize their life experiences in practical ways for living healthy, successful, and creative lives. Eleanor strongly believes that each individual's core Self manifests fully when given support and encouragement. She also believes that many people simply need directional help to feel empowered in their lives. Eleanor and Marvin work together in documenting **Noble Energy Wellness Tools**™. They met in India on August 13, 1978 and have been married since 1979. They live closely together with their cats and dogs. They very much enjoy their children and grandchildren.

Eleanor has served as President of the Southern California Society for Clinical Hypnosis from 2010 to 2013. She is an American Society of Clinical Hypnosis (ASCH) approved consultant, a founding member of the Erickson Institute Los Angeles, a certified Clean Language Coach (Institute for Leadership Management), and a Professional and Board Certified Coach. She is also a member of numerous other professional organizations.

COLLABORATIVE ASSISTANCE

Marvin M. Portner, Ph.D.

Marvin Portner, M.D. had been doing healing work for many years when Eleanor introduced him to Reiki in 1978. The purity and the healing power of the Reiki energy impressed him. Marvin found that the intensity and reliability of the energy work he did after his Reiki initiations brought a new dimension to his other work with patients. He expanded his study of Reiki through the years and has been consistently using and teaching it since he and Eleanor were initiated as Reiki Master Teachers in 1982.

Marvin M. Portner, M.D., was born in Detroit, Michigan on March 15.. He is Board Certified in Internal Medicine, Allergy, and Immunology, both Pediatric and Adult. Marvin graduated from the University of Michigan Medical School with high honors. Although Marvin worked in traditional medicine for many years, he became an early pioneer in the field of Holistic Integratted Medicine. He has been involved in synthesizing/integrating Western and Eastern medicine as well as working with mind/body medicine for over thirty-five years. His medical practice remains personalized and interactive, making him a rare practitioner in today's marketplace. Marvin practices as a medical consultant. He holds medical licenses in both California and in South Carolina.

Cindy Smith

Cindy Smith was introduced to First and Second Degree Reiki by Eleanor. In 2008 she was initiated as a Reiki Master by Eleanor and Marvin. Upon learning Reiki, Cindy began working with the Noble Energy Wellness tools and found them profoundly expansive in her own development. She and Eleanor began working together on developing the Reiki Mind Maps that serve as a highly instructive tool in learning and using the tools taught in all levels of Reiki. Cindy is an avid student of philosophy and mysticism. She began working intensively with Noble Sciences™ Tools and collaborates with Eleanor in further developing her materials. Cindy met her husband through a mutual love of skydiving. They have been married for 35 years and have one child. Cindy has a Master of Science in Information Systems and Technology Management.

Important Note:

Through the years many factions developed in the Reiki organization and individuals began to change the attunements and the teaching, thus, diluting its energy and dissipating its integrity. Not all individuals who claim to teach Reiki have the keys to do the attunements and some people who claim to teach Reiki do not even realize that a specific attunement process that sets the energy path is required. Eleanor and Marvin, continue to honor the purity of the Usui Reiki teaching and do the Usui Reiki attunements without any modifications to the system.

♦ ♦ ♦

Classes

Reiki First Degree, Second Degree and Third Degree (part 1 and 2) trainings are available.

For more information call:
Portner Medical Corporation at: (310) 266-3050 or
Noble Sciences Sacred Synthesis, LLC. at: (310) 403-4347 or contact the office at: info@noblesciences.com.

For information about training or coaching using Reiki contact Eleanor at: ehp@noblesciences.com or call her at: (310) 403-4347.

Noble Energy Wellness™

Noble Energy Wellness focuses on Energy Medicine and Holistic options for healing and health. Dr. Marvin and Dr. Eleanor teach energy wellness in their weekly Manifest Your Dreams Webinar. Through the webinar, you can learn how to live authentically while manifesting your actual potential by understanding and integrating the Four Worlds into your daily life. Register to learn how you can manifest your dreams by attending these weekly webinars.
https://nobleenergywellness.com

Noble Energy Maps™

Noble Energy Maps focus on Dr. Eleanor's proprietary and innovative system for mapping how cosmic energy impacted you during your childhood development and how you can use this knowledge to optimally time your decisions, identify your life purpose, and live a self-realized life. Dr. Eleanor statistically validated her system through over 45,000 cases and uses Noble Energy Maps to guide clients toward wholeness and empowerment.
https://www.nobleenergywellness.com/energy-map/

The Noble Logo has a special place in Dr. Eleanor's heart. Her first cat, **Noble**, lived to age 22 and was an inspiration and guide during important times in Dr. Eleanor's growth and studies. He worked with her and Dr. Marvin when they hosted weekend groups for over ten years. Noble always helped guide them toward whom to work with next, as well as to the area that clients needed to work on. Dr. Eleanor uses calculations based on research done on her two homegrown twin kittens. The critical human developmental times used in Dr. Eleanor's proprietary maps, have proven accurate clinically and statistically, which map the Four Worlds in your energy field and how you can best function.

The Mandala of Synthesis describes the elements coded into Dr. Eleanor's proprietary Noble Energy Maps. The Mandala of Synthesis includes the Kabbalistic Tree of Life, Chakras, Astrology, the Hexagrams of the I-Ching, and critical times in early Human Development. Dr. Eleanor calculates her maps and integrates the information coded into a graphic illustrating the way you use your energy, where the flow of energy becomes clear. Dr. Eleanor's extensive education as a social scientist, researcher, and clinician has empowered her to formulate a complete system that recognizes the complexity of your consciousness and shows how you can best use it for growth and expansion of consciousness.

https://www.nobleenergywellness.com/mandala-of-synthesis

www.ingramcontent.com/pod-product-compliance
Lightning Source LLC
Chambersburg PA
CBHW070104080526
44586CB00013B/1182